AF237284

Katrin Rabe
Silk – Inner strength and outer protection

Katrin Rabe

Silk

Inner strength and outer protection

The homeopathic remedy Sericum coconum

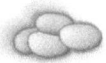

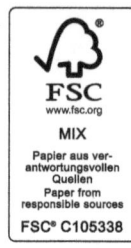

Bibliographical information of the German National Library
The German National Library indexes this publication in the German National Bibliography; detailed bibliographical information may be obtained on the internet at https://www.dnb.de/en.

Copy and design: Katrin Rabe

English language: Andre Rabe

Print and publishing
BoD – Books on Demand, Norderstedt

ISBN: 978-3-754-34590-0

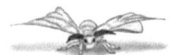

Heartfelt thanks to
Renate Siefert;
She showed me the world of
resonant trituration.

Sincere thanks to all
participants of the trituration and remedy self-experience.
You all have contributed valuable information
to the emergence of
Silk – Sericum coconicum's
Remedy make-up.

Loving thanks especially
to the entity Silk.
It gives me strength and protection
on my path.

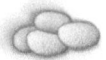

Table of contents

My journey to the remedy silk

Ever from a young age I've had a strong urge to travel to China. I didn't know why, but I dreamt peculiar dreams of living there. These dreams were particularly vivid and surprising. They couldn't even be explained as a by-product of television programming, as my family didn't own a TV set at this time.

At the age of about 10 I developed an interest in Chinese art. I went to any exhibition that had even the slightest to do with the subject. Using my pocket money, I bought books from antiquarian bookshops about Chinese painting. These books I would then pore over for hours on end. I tried to replicate the art of Chinese painting by copying the pictures.

Around the age of 14 I was gifted a silk cloth. I may not have liked the color very much, but it just felt magnificent. No itching or scratching of the skin, simply soft and warm. This was what gave my dream journey to China a concrete shape – the silk. Painting on silk first became a hobby and later on, for a few years, my job.

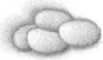

My homeopathic meeting with silk occurred after a minor accident, in the course of which I severely rolled my right ankle and partially tore a tendon in there. Acute treatment was undertaken with *Arnica montana C10,000* directly on-site, which managed to dampen the pain to a mostly acceptable level and softened the shock.

Homeopathic after-treatment was carried out with *Bellis perennis* and *Ruta graveolens* in various potencies. These had usually produced good results in similar circumstances. This time, however, neither the pain, nor the swelling nor the over-articulation of the ankle went away. Even after two weeks I was unable to walk without pain, which went counter to all my experiences with homeopathic treatment.

For this reason, I began to look for a better remedy for myself. My thoughts soon fell on silk. I love silk and it has qualities (see ch. "Qualities") that have much in common with tissues found in our bodies, such as skin, tendons and ligaments. Since I like to experiment, I produced and ingested the homeopathic remedy Silk in a potency of C10,000 using a radionic instrument.

What happened then was simply incredible! Within a day, pain and swelling had completely gone. Just a week later, both full stability and normal mobility of the joint had been restored.

This accident was over 15 years ago and in all that time I have never had an injury of the same kind, even though this used to be the case about once or twice a year before I started taking Silk.

Apart from the compelling effect the remedy had in this emergency situation, the remedy's other positive effects for psyche and physical health gradually emerged. In the chapter "My first experiences with silk" I have written down the most important points of my notes. These notes provided the foundation for my further work with this homeopathic remedy.

After this positive experience my interest in silk was significantly stoked, especially as it was not yet available as a remedy. After encouragement from homeopath Renate Siefert, who, along with Frans Vermeulen, has supported my homeopathic development and training in extraordinary ways, I undertook a C4 trituration of untreated silk fibers with other homeopaths and interested lay people.

This personal encounter with Silk yielded much valuable information that proved instrumental for the further development of the remedy silk cocoon and its use in homeopathic practice. (see ch. "Text passages from the trituration protocols")

Having been fortunate enough to witness several positive treatments in my own practice, I also initiated a self-experience of this remedy. The results of this experience, of which six persons partook, are also mentioned in this book.

I'm glad that my journey to the remedy Silk has reached its first goal in the publication of this book. I hope that this publication will help you to use Silk (*Sericum coconum*) to great effect in your homeopathic practice.

Sincerely,
Katrin Rabe

A brief history of silk

Discovery

The discovery of silk is shrouded in myth. One of the most well-known legends is the following:

Around 2640 BC, Si-Ling-Chi, the wife of Chinese emperor Huangdi, supposedly strolled through the gardens. A silk cocoon then fell into her tea cup. When she removed it, the cocoon's thread unraveled, leaving her with shining strings instead of the cocoon in her hands.

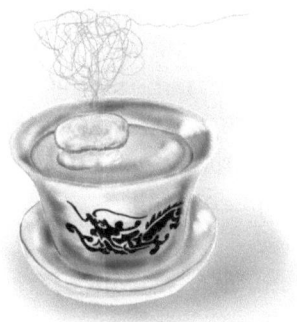

This delighted the young empress so much that she collected 1,000 cocoons and used them to weave a cloak for the emperor.

In her honor, the thread was named "Si", upon which most modern names are based. (English: silk, German: Seide, Swedish: silke, Japanese: seri, Latin: sericum)

For emperors and kings

The manufacture of silk is very laborious, which ensured that this precious material was initially only available to the Chinese emperor and his wives. Only around 1,200 BC this privilege was extended to aristocrats and rich merchants.
Circa 300 BC it was permitted to teach the process of silk-making at the Japanese Imperial Court. Much later, silk found its way over the famous Silk Road to European monarchs. However, because of the long and perilous journey on the Silk Road, silk was prohibitively expensive and many sought ways to produce it in Europe, as well.

Secrets and industrial espionage

The manufacture of silk was a jealously guarded secret. Because of the threat of capital punishment, it took over two and a half millennia until the secret was revealed and the making of silk became known outside of China's borders.

The first step was teaching the process at the Japanese Imperial Court. The fact that this knowledge reached Europe is thanks to possibly the first ever case of industrial espionage.

Two Nestorian monks, sent by emperor Justinian around 555 AD, supposedly managed to smuggle seeds of the Mulberry tree and Bombyx eggs to Constantinople in their walking sticks.

This marked the beginning of silk production in the rest of Asia, Europe and, finally, in America as well.

The manufacture of silk

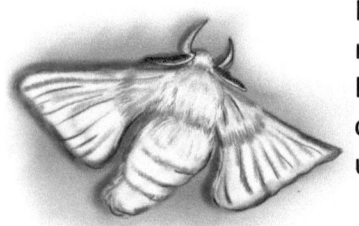

By far the most widely used silkworm moth is the domestic silkworm, Bombyx mori. This moth has been cultivated for millennia and is now unable to survive in the wild.

Other moths also produce silk, but far smaller quantities and of lesser quality than Bombyx mori. The cultivation of silkworm moths is very delicate. Exacting climatic circumstances, precise feeding and good hygiene must be observed throughout, as these determine the quality of the produced silk. Furthermore, silkworms are susceptible to bacterial illnesses.

The female lays around 500 eggs and dies thereafter. The eggs are oval, flat and about 1 to 1.5 mm long. The fertilized eggs endure the winter and the silkworms hatch the following spring.

In modern silk manufacture, various methods are employed to produce several crops a year.

After hatching, the silkworm will eat around 25g of mulberry leaves every day of its around 30 days of growth.

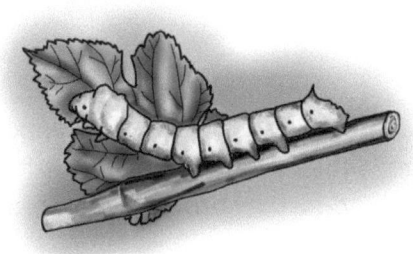

During this process, it will increase its weight by a factor of 8,000.

After this, it stops eating and begins to spin a cocoon for itself.

In this process, every silkworm produces a silk thread around 400 to 900 meters in length using its two silk glands. This equates to one or two grams of raw silk. After finishing the cocoons, the silkworm becomes a pupa. It remains in this stadium for 8-12 days in its silken cocoon which forms an effective protection against outer influences.

After this time, its metamorphosis to a moth is complete. It will then secrete a fluid which dissolves the cocoon in one spot, thereby destroying the long thread of silk. The pieces of such destroyed cocoons can only be used for very poor-quality silk.

To combat this, the pupae are killed by way of heat or boiling before reaching this stadium, to prevent them hatching and thus destroying the silk thread.

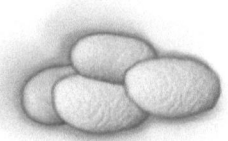

Boiling has the added benefit of dissolving the silk gum which glues the thread together and lends the cocoon its stability. After this, one can unravel the cocoons and further process the thread for spinning and weaving.

For spinning, several silk threads measuring an astonishing several hundred meters in length (compare to cotton at 15~56mm) are plied together, depending on the desired yarn weight.

Composition and qualities

Silk is the secretion of a silkworm's silk glands, which it uses to spin a cocoon. It is liquid on secretion and hardens upon air contact.

Composition

A single silk thread consists of two silk fibers (Fibroin) which are surrounded by silk gum (Sericin, silk glue), also called silk filament.

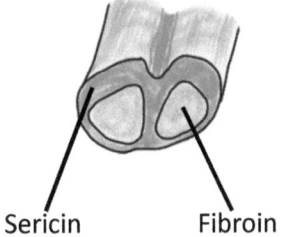

Sericin   Fibroin

The silk filament makes up about 70-80% of the thread. Fibroin is a Sulphur-free, highly polymeric protein, that is to say it is a naturally occurring polyamide fiber. The recurring patterns of amino acids give silk its shine, softness and elasticity.

The amount of silk gum (Sericin) in a silk thread is between 20-30%.

The Sericin holds the cocoon together, meaning it sticks the fibers together and so gives the cocoon stability and longevity.

Other components of silk are 1.2 to 1.6% carbohydrates, 0.7% organic components and 0.2% natural dyes.

Qualities

The real duty of the silk thread is the protection of the moth's becoming and growth. To ensure success at this venture, silk is endowed with important and unique qualities. It is soft, protects from heat and cold, can absorb moisture and release it again and has high tensile strength. It can only be attacked by few substances, which gives it great longevity. These and further special properties elevate silk above other natural fibers.

Some facts and stats:
- Silk is one of the lightest natural fibers with a density of only around 1.25 g/cm^3
- To produce 1 kg raw silk, 5-10 kg of cocoons are processed, depending on quality. This equates to around two to six thousand cocoons.
- The weight unit for silk is 1 Momme = 1 Pongé = 4.306 g/m^2.

- Despite its fiber thickness of only 12-25 μm it has a greater breaking length (that is the length at which a fiber breaks under its own weight) than steel.
- Its tensile strength is 350 MPa, which means that it is possible to suspend a load of 3.56 metric tons from a silk rope with a cross sectional area of only 1 cm². The only known natural fiber that is stronger is spider silk, with up to 25 tons/cm²

Other important features that make silk especially important to the textile industry are the following:
- A high ductility. A silk thread of 1 m length can stretch up to 15 cm without breaking.
- High moisture absorption. Silk can absorb 30% of its weight in moisture without feeling wet.
- Great skin tolerability. Because of its organic nature, it lets the skin breathe and feels stimulating.
- It is a good insulation against heat, cold and electricity.
- Silk is very easily dyed.
- Low flammability. Its flash point is at 171 °C. It also suffocates the flame because of carbon buildup that is a product of its burning.

All this makes silk a very stable and long-lasting material that hardly rots or otherwise degenerates.

Care

Silk is a very long-lasting textile, if one keeps to certain basic rules:

- Use only enzyme free detergents (natural soaps, wool detergent). Because silk is made of natural protein structures, the enzymes in regular detergent would slowly dissolve it over time.
- Protect your silk from direct sunlight, as too much sunlight will cause it to bleach and yellow.
- Never tumble dry silk clothing, as this will make it shrink strongly.
- Don't wring silk after the wash.
- Iron silk while it's slightly moist.

Applications of silk

Textile industry

Because of its special qualities, silk has many use cases. The largest of these is the textile industry. Features like shine, soft fall, lightness of the fabric, good color absorption, skin tolerability and stretchiness are important for silk's usage for luxurious clothing such as underwear, festive dress, socks, but also bed linens and so on.

Military and sports

Silk's extraordinary strength as a fabric because of its fiber length has led to its use for military applications. Supposedly, it was used by the Mongol hordes as part of protective clothing, where it, combined with leather and iron, was very hard to penetrate with arrows. But even modern militaries and competitive sports use silk (mainly as underwear) for its good insulation capability.

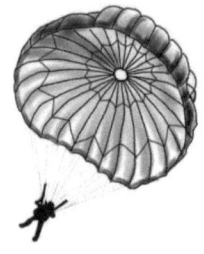 Silk production was introduced in Germany to make parachutes for the military. Besides that, it was also used to smuggle secret maps and notes. These would be written down onto silk sheets, as they can be folded down to very small sizes and thus more easily concealed.

Medicine

Another area of use for silk is in medicine. Because silk doesn't decompose in the body, silk thread was used for stitches to close internal and external wounds. In vascular surgery, silk hose has been used to replace damaged blood vessels. For this purpose, it has largely been replaced by synthetic materials, however.

Cosmetics

Recently, silk in the form of silk proteins has started to take over the cosmetics industry as well. There, they utilize features such as its good moisture absorption, skin tolerability and the famous silk shine.

Arts

Even in arts, silk has a steady place. As a base for calligraphy, silk paintings or in fine silk embroidery, it entrances the viewer with its delicacy and its strong, clear colors. As strings in traditional Asian musical instruments, it lends them their inimitable sound.

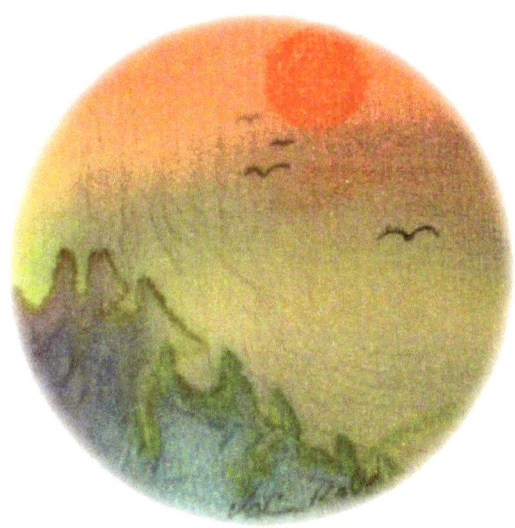

Silk in daily language

In German, the expression **"halbseiden"** (literally half-silken, meaning shady) is often used to refer to people that seem dubious or questionable for any reason. At the creation of this expression, only very few people could afford the luxury of dressing in silk garments. Therefore, this adjective refers to people (especially women), who would associate with the "higher" echelons of society, without really belonging to them.

"Soft as silk, silky smooth, silky matt" are adjectives that refer to certain features of silk and are used to highlight special features of other materials (textiles, hair, colors, skin, ...).
These words are designed to make a material appear more valuable than it actually is. This often happens with textiles, when marketing advertises so called "artificial silks".

To be dressed **"in silks and satins"** means to live in great wealth, but also means that someone is a boaster, a show-off. The expression is also used to signify that something is especially precious. Both these fabrics are very valuable, as they are laborious to make, and could therefore only be worn by rulers and aristocrats in the past.

To **"hang by a (silk) thread"** signifies an uncertain situation that may well end badly. This possibly refers to the make-up of the very thin, and therefore seemingly weak silk thread. Another possible explanation is a reference to the goddesses of fate, that spin the thread of destiny, or the Sword of Damocles of Greek myth, which hung above him from only a silk thread (hair of a horse's tail), to remind him of the danger he faced.

My first experiences with Silk

After taking the remedy Silk C10,000, produced with a radionic device from thread of an undyed Chinese silk sheet, apart from the previously mentioned quick healing of the ankle joint, several other positive developments started in my life. These clearly showed the powerful potential of Silk as a homeopathic remedy.

Here are the most important themes:

Decisiveness

I just cannot decide which professional path to take. Should I continue to be an employee or dare to take step to being a homeopathic healer with my own practice. These and other thoughts often cross my mind, especially in connection with the accident in which I hurt my ankle. About a month after taking the remedy I now have clarity; I quit my job and open my own practice.

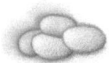

Inner strength

I feel very strong inside, I can get my way without conflict, yelling or similar. Someone compliments me on this: "I have never met someone who can reach their goals in such a gentle yet firm way."

Confidence

I haven't felt this good and confident in a long time. I'm happy, almost exuberant, and simply enjoy life. I laugh more often.

Travel

Very excited ahead of every journey, preparations were made very early, everything was organized exactly, especially when journeying further away or abroad. I could hardly sleep the night before, would often wake during the night and get up very early on the day. Since taking silk I'm much more relaxed ahead of travel.

Fear of something happening on the journey

Fear that something might happen. On car rides, I was unable to relax as a passenger, couldn't sleep, even when I trusted the driver, since taking the remedy I am able to sleep on car rides.

Dreams of travelling to China

I am travelling to China by train.

In another time period, I wander alone through China.

I want to travel to China, but miss the train or am unable to buy the ticket. These dreams have not reoccurred since taking Silk.

Sunlight

My sensitivity to sunlight has strongly diminished. I can enjoy the sunlight on my face, when I used to try to always keep my face shaded. Even my eyes are less sensitive to brightness, I can enjoy a walk in the sun without squinting. Since taking the remedy, I am better able to endure the heat in the sun.

Silk clothing

I have always enjoyed wearing silk, but I think I do even more so now. If I could afford it, I would probably only wear silk garments. I just feel good in them.

Skin

My skin, especially on the legs, the hands and the face were unbearably dry. After every bit of contact with water, especially chlorinated water at the pool or soapy water from bathing, I needed to generously apply lotion to keep from itching. Dust, sand and wool would itch too and exacerbate the dryness.

After taking Silk my skin takes on a healthier look. The regulation of my skin's moisture levels normalizes within a month. Since then, applying moisturizing lotion is only really necessary e.g., after swimming in chlorinated water. Normal showering and bathing now no longer leads to itchiness or skin dryness.

Hair

Hair was very dry, without shine, plain. They would quickly attract a static charge, e.g., while combing them, which effect disappeared within four weeks of remediation with Silk. The hair now grows without breaking, has more shine and is curlier, which matches the way it used to be in my childhood.

The individual hairs are very thin and have the interesting quality of being able to stretch quite far without breaking. (This elasticity is still present, so it might be a special feature that may indicate Silk.)

Tendon injury

Outside of right foot, from slipping on the stairs, strong pain, great swelling and hypermobility of the joint, the symptoms improving very rapidly. Within 12 hours, pain and swelling are gone, which had previously been unsuccessfully treated with *Arnica montana*, *Ruta graveolens* and *Bellis perennis*.

Within the week, the joint's normal mobility has been restored. Although I used to fall victim to these types of injuries often in the past, it has since never happened again.

Travel sickness

Nausea all the way to vomiting, while travelling by car, bus, tram, plane or on a ship. Train journeys present no problems.

Better:	fresh air; concentrating on the road ahead
Worse:	Fuel smell; curvy road; waves

Since treatment with Silk, most of these complaints have gone away. Under extreme conditions such as travelling by bus on curvy roads while it stinks of diesel, nausea may still appear, but vomiting so far has not.

C4 - trituration as a valuable source of information

Trituration is the way of producing a homeopathic remedy practiced and taught by Samuel Hahnemann.

Sensitive homeopaths have discovered, that everything we feel from stage to stage during trituration has to do with the spirit and the character of whichever substance we are preparing. While we calmly and patiently rub, we enter the territory, in a manner of speaking, of this substance, for instance a plant or mineral, and we are able to physically, psychically and spiritually experience its features and its being.

If we write all this down, we get a trituration protocol that reflects our own experiences with the substance. If we summarize what we've experienced in a group setting, we will discover that although the individual impressions of participants will vary, they will nonetheless touch upon similar themes. Thereby a picture of the substance in many facets is produced.

Hahnemann advocated for each homeopath to produce their own remedies. He was surely aware of the deep experience and insight this process triggers in us. And he must have known that the process connected us to the spirit of the remedy in a very particular way.

Resonant trituration to the 4th level is especially suited to gaining a deep understanding of the healing powers and the spirit of our triturated substance. During trituration we follow along with the substance on the steps of healing and accompany it on the way to the "healed healer". With all our senses, we experience the original pain, the recognition of the inherent power and lastly the freeing of healing power.

In my experience, this allows us to internalize and recognize the therapeutic possibilities of the remedy. A resonant trituration (C4 trituration) strengthens our powers of perception especially well.

The process of trituration is extensively described in the book "Der Weg der Homöopathie" by Renate Siefert. Using several trituration protocols as examples, she explains, why trituration, that is to say the process of energizing, are the key to a homeopathic remedy's healing potential.

The homeopathic remedy *Sericum coconum* is described in that book with a complete trituration protocol by Renate Siefert.

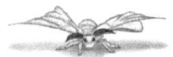

C4 trituration of some threads of an untreated silk cocoon

On 04/26/2008 six persons (five females, one male) triturated silk in Vallentuna, Sweden. They utilized the outer threads of two silk cocoons from the domestic silkworm Bombyx mori. These cocoons originated in China and were graciously provided by Plauener Spinnhütte of Plauen, Germany.

The participants were aware of the material used for the trituration. This seminar's purpose was first and foremost to familiarize them with C4 trituration. As a C4 trituration is a very personal experience, the protocols will not be reproduced in their entireties, but only certain excerpts, which the participants agreed to have published.

Two of the participants did not write revelatory protocols and as such, only their observations in the summary following the trituration will be used to strengthen the messages received by the other participants.

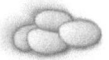

GDV bio-energy field analysis for the documentation of energetic processes

The energetic influence of the trituration process of silk on the participants was documented with GDV bio-energy field imaging. This technique enables us to measure changes in fine material and energetic areas, before these changes can affect the appearance or disappearance of symptoms that are perceptible to us. Because this event was the first trituration where such documentation techniques were used, only possible conclusions can be drawn from the results in this publication.

Measurements were taken of each participant the day before trituration, minutes before the start of trituration and directly afterwards. Measurements were taken by a person that did not take part in the seminar and had no prior knowledge of participants' medical history.

Text passages from the trituration protocols

I would like to begin with a few passages from level C4. On this level, the being Silk comes to us. It speaks to us as a "healed healer" and gives us a direct insight into its power and its healing potential.

The message of Silk, as rendered by person 1

Silky smooth
Soft and delicate,
mellow and empathetic,
compassionate is my heart.
I protect the delicate.
I protect the growing.
Warmth courses through my whole body.
I warm.

My love I give to you.
My protection, my strength I give to you.
I do not want to know your doubts,
for you do not need them.
Take the next step.

Life is full of lightness.
A home,
you build yourself your home.
Fortune,
you have all you need.

Believe in your power.
You reach your goal.
Make a decision.
Be clear and precise.

Everything feels easy.
Doing is ease,
when it comes from within.

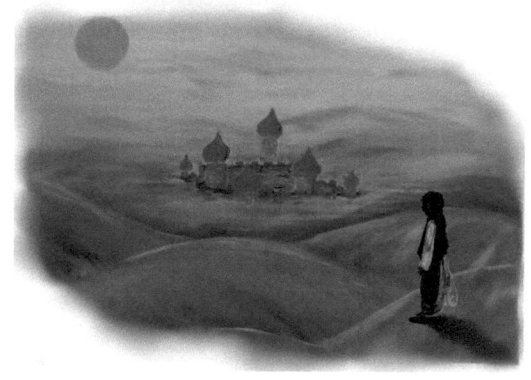

The message of Silk, as rendered by person 2

I am the spirit of Silk.
Invisible almost
and without outer illusion.
I know no violence,
give sure footing to the weak.
Bind the powers into one.
I give you power and inner peace,
the calm of humility
and the still shine
of inner strength.

So, we go together
with the caravan eastward,
where the light appears
on the horizon.

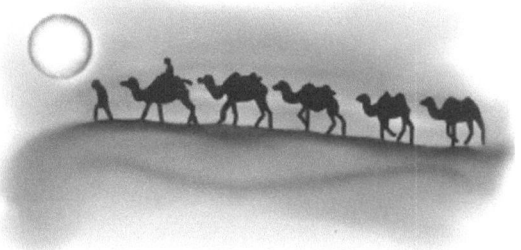

And every day comes new
in its own beauty.

See, they appreciate my shine,
my splendor,
my appearance.

Don't let yourself be blinded.
You have known me deeper.
Take my hand,
I am with you.

The message of Silk, as rendered by person 3

Be pure and delicate with yourself.

Lightness	Happiness	Eternity
Forever	Pease	Rest
Young	Soft	Sleep

I awaken creativity.
I awaken patience.
I can help women get pregnant.
Children get security from me.

"With all peace and harmony" or "the creative making"
– are the two ways to use silk.

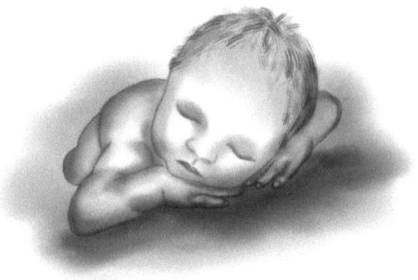

Silk's impression on person 4

Everything is good now.
Can start anew without destruction.
Can start over and take with me what is important to me.
Calm rises.
Want to take everything more as it comes,
not always change and improve.
What is, is good.
Self-assurance.

Someone stands above me, guards and protects me.

Someone holds their hand over me.

Pure silk purifies life.

.

Summary of the themes of the trituration

The following is a summary of the themes of Silk that emerged during this trituration. Several of these themes have been corroborated by successful treatment with the remedy.

Threads, strings

Feeling like a thread being pulled from the forehead. (P1)
Hanging on threads and freeing oneself from these threads. (P1)
Endless thread, spinning, weaving. (P2)
Seeing a blue thread in the lactose. (P5)

Freedom, life, theater

Life is a play; Pinocchio, hanging on threads and freeing oneself from these threads; freedom to live your life. (P1)
I show the way to freedom; parents protect and show the way to life. (P1)
Here I am and I feel free. (P2)
Life is eternal art and you are your own artist; create your own life. (P3)

Wish for child, pregnancy

Warmth, like from a baby. (P1)
I can help women get pregnant. (P3)

Travel, efforts on a travel, not giving up

It's a long road. (P1)
Caravan, the silk balls are moving in a row like camels. (P1)
China, travelling to China. (P1)
Eyes closing, weary from the long journey. (P1)
I want to stay, no - do not stop, go on, on, on... (P1)
Mustn't close my eyes or I will fall asleep, must not lose sight of
the goal. (P1)
Be patient, don't give up, show no weakness, find shelter like on
a journey. (P2)
The caravan moves on into the unknown, wandering. (P2)
A long way to learn to see, to shape, to get to know oneself. (P3)
A long journey, together. (P3)
No-one can stop me, slowly I reach my goal, as slowly as a snail, a
strong snail, totally reliable. (P4)
Pause has taken away the rhythm, will I find the way back? (P4)
Hiking through the wilderness to the big sea. (P4

Beauty

At the end there is beauty no-one dares to destroy. (P2)
A seductive, beautiful woman. (P3)
Silk is the being of beauty; it clothes the gods. (Aphrodite, Hercules) (P3)
Like a flower, blue and beautiful. (P4)
Thinking of beautiful places, nature, fields and meadows. (P4)

Protection/Lack of protection, delicate, fragile

Nothing can hurt me. (P1)
Protection, I protect the butterfly. (P1)
I am protected in a cocoon of pure light, silk envelops me. (P1)
Being taken care of, kept like a treasure. (P1)
Silky smooth, soft and delicate, sensitive and empathic, compassionate is my heart, I protect the delicate,
I protect the growth. (P1)
I will give protection to the defenseless. (P2)
Children gain protection from this remedy. (P3)
Not wanting to hurt, soft as silk, vulnerable and delicate. (P4)
Someone watches over me, guards and protects me. (P4)
Thinking of my son, he is so easily vulnerable. (P5)

Longing, sadness

Strong longing, tears welling up, sadness. (P1)
Waving goodbye, mourning, I miss her soothing voice. (P4)

Strength – Gentleness

Soft and gentle, delicate. (P1)
Strong together. (P1)
I have nothing but my strength that resists any stress test. (P2)
We have no haste, we save our strength, together we are strong.
(P2)
Victory through silent strength. (P2)
Self-assured, strong integrity, power in itself. (P3)
Being different is strong as well. (P4)
A strong snail, totally reliable, carries others far. (P4)

Stillness, silence, inner voice

I hear nothing around me. (P1)
It should be silent, stillness should overpower the outside noise,
listen to the voice from within. (P1)
Stillness is around, and loneliness. (P2)
The silent shine of inner strength. (P2)
All noises disturb me, sensitive to noise, I can feel their
scratching in my teeth. (P3)
Sensitive to sound. (P4)

Immortality, endlessness

Dreaming, the endlessness, jumping into the chasm like in the
movie "Crouching Tiger, Hidden Dragon". (P1)
I rub endlessly, I want to rub like the symbol of infinity. (P1)
The string, endless. (P2)
At the end there is beauty no-one dares to destroy. (P2)
The font of youth is in silk and in us, it only has to be awakened.
(P3)
I feel old and young at the same time. (P4)

Transformation, development, metamorphosis

Transformation, the butterfly rises. (P1)
Development to enjoyment of life. (P1)
Gather strength for the new beginning, being there, being strong, being ready. (P2)
Accepting death as a way of transformation to a new kind of being. (P2)
All the colors of the rainbow are hidden within silk, you can set them free. (P3)
I want vitality, just jump in and swim, five days, then everything will be better; to part from this old life?
No, part from myself, from my dark side that is always holding me back. (P4)

Warmth

I'm getting warm, I'm getting hot. (P1)
I feel warmth. (P1)
The heat bothers me, warmth is a theme of silk. (P1)
Warmth courses through my entire body, I warm. (P1)
Warmth like from a baby. (P1)
I'm feeling hot, a cool silk blouse would be nice now. (P3)
It's getting warmer. (P4)

Knowledge, secrecy

I know too much; knowledge gets in my way. (P1)
I feel light, without thought, without knowledge. (P2)
Working in secrecy. (P2)
Diving into the depth of my own self, to find answers. (P3)

Future, confidence, ease

Left, rubbing with ease with the left, with the left = with ease.
(P1)
Thinking of the future, the heart fills with assurance. (P1)
Your doubts, you need them not. (P1)
Believe in your power, you will reach your goal. (P1)
Everything feels light. (P1)
Doing is easy, when it comes from within. (P1)
Wherever we're going, we'll get there. (P2)
I feel light, without thought, without knowledge. (P2)
In me are assurance and happiness; I know the direction,
I go on. (P2)
I feel light as a silk thread. (P3)
Everything is good, I am good as I am, finally I am doing
something for myself, a good feeling. (P4)

Coherence, effort, resistance

It is incredible how tightly the threads stick together. (P1)
Effort to break apart the bundle. (P1)
Resistance, I feel the silk resisting, defying the trituration. (P1)
The silk is resisting, the threads are helping each other, sticking together. (P1)
It clumps together, it finds itself, the resistance of the weak. (P2)
We stick together, we find one another. (P2)
We all are bound together by a single thread, thin and strong. (P3)
Silk ball too large. (P4)
Effort, thumb hurting. (P4)
Difficult to break apart the silk, what a tenacious material. (P5)
Feeling of harmony and belonging together; society. (P5)

(P1) – (P5) stand in for the various participants in the trituration. These numbers were listed to highlight the similar experiences participants had.

Summary of the GDV bio-energy field scans

All participants, save for number 4, reacted to the trituration with a balancing of and improvement to their emotional-energetic reaction potential. Especially where liver, kidneys and the right cardiac area were concerned, there was a positive impact of the unit of trituration process and silk cocoon's energetic effect.

Depending on individual inclinations, we were able to see effects in the following areas: breasts, pulmonary organs, gall bladder, spleen, pituitary gland and thyroid.

Person 4 displayed a considerably worse energetic image directly after the seminar. The areas of: kidneys, gall bladder, back and sinuses as well as the thyroid and pituitary glands reacted with a drastic decline of their energetic state.

For this reason, the participant was measured again the following day. The measurements now showed an improvement and a balancing, above and beyond their original state, before the seminar. This is indicative of the trituration of silk cocoon having a healing impact on the participant.

The directly visible energetic decline may correspond to the first reaction upon taking a new homeopathic remedy, the improvement the following day is already the first positive step toward healing, which is also partly visible from participant 4's listed quotes.

The measured results can be displayed by way of various graphs. For reasons of clarity, this publication only contains a depiction of person 4's average reaction potential.

Further images can be viewed at my internet site www.gesund-mit-homöopathie.de (at C4 Verreibungen/Seide)

Summary of the GDV bio-energy field scans for participant 4

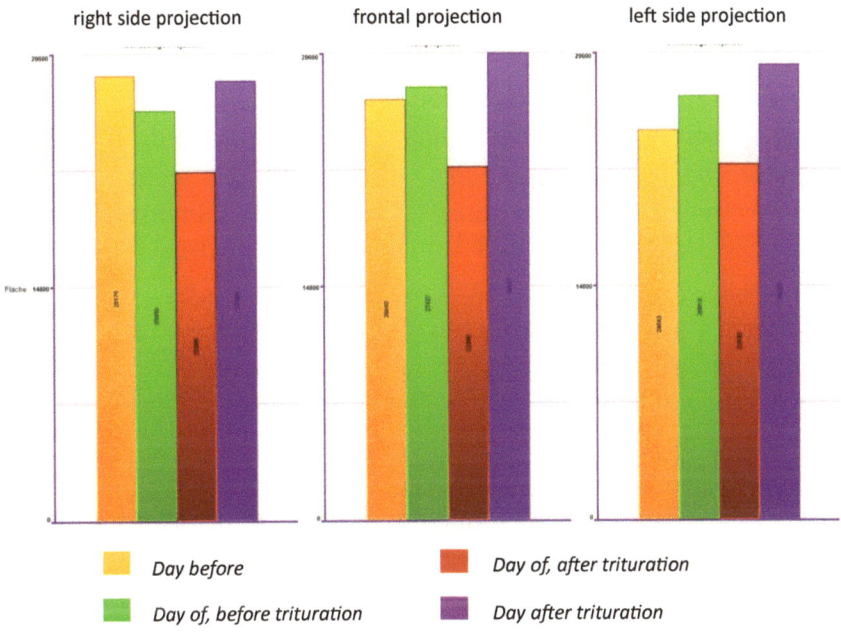

The bar charts show the decline directly after trituration (red bar) and the improvement of their reaction potential (purple bar) of the whole organism even above and beyond their potential of the day before. It also shows a balancing of between the right and left body halves, which already took place during trituration.

Homeopathic remedy self-experience (proving)

Execution

In November 2016 six participants took part in a homeopathic remedy self-experience (proving) with the remedy *Sericum coconum bombyx mori (ser-coc)*. The participants were not told which remedy they were taking. They were only told this after the proving's conclusion.

The participants were instructed to begin taking the globules on a day convenient to them and to take note of the time and day they began. They were also instructed to begin notation 3 days prior to first taking the remedy.

Ingestion was to take place once a day, until first reactions were to be observed. Independently of the manifestation of any symptoms, ingestion was to be ended after one week at maximum. After taking the remedy the final time, observation was kept up for another four to six weeks. Three participants took part in regular interviews, the others provided their notes after ending the proving.

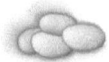

Two further people were sent the remedy, but did not take them and therefore also provided no notes.

The specific potency used was *Sericum coconum C30*, produced by Enzian-Apotheke in Munich, Germany. (s. address data at the end of this book)

Participants

Person 1 (P1) – Female, 41 years
Person 2 (P2) – Female, 36 years
Person 3 (P3) – Male, 37 years
Person 4 (P4) – Male, 45 years
Person 5 (P5) – Female, 45 years
Person 6 (P6) – Female, 55 years

Peculiarities, as noted by myself

Dates

It was rather difficult to set dates with the participants for their personal interviews. Agreed-upon dates were often postponed or simply not kept.

Something gets lost during the journey

Participant 6's notes were nowhere to be found. No record exists of them, neither in her nor in my computer. This reminded me of the unpredictability of a journey, as one often relates to silk. In the times of the silk road, only part of the valuably freight would often arrive at their destination.

For this reason, only some parts of the participant's notes, which she still remembered, are listed here.

Decisions are made, a new journey begins

In the life of person 7, who did not take the remedy and didn't take any notes, I was nonetheless able to observe some important changes. During the proving, she left her significantly older partner and after much back and forth finally dared to take the step and move into her own apartment. She seemed much calmer and more self-confident.

A step is not taken

Person 8 never began the proving. She was afraid of not being healthy enough to take part. Upon inquiry, she stated several time that she was now willing to start. However, she never took this final step.

Themes of the proving

Communication/contact

Good mood and very communicative, meeting people. (P1)

Heightened desire to communicate. (P1)

Flirted a lot, while feeling: "Oh, I'm interesting". (P2)

I also avoid talking a lot and conversations. (P2)

Excited and happy thoughts about meeting new people. (P5)

People (taxi drivers, neighbors, colleagues) are suddenly even more open and trusting of me. (P5)

Departure, decision-making

Desire to express myself more clearly, be more visible and audible. (P1)

Plans for developing the practice. (P1)

It is time to live more outward and forward. Many ideas and some plans are already manifesting, the sleeves are rolled up. (P1)

I'm on the road again. Where to, I don't yet know. Many things appeal to me, but I don't have a clear direction yet. (unsatisfied with current work situation) (P2)

I want to proceed at my own speed. I feel a resistance to tempo dictated by other. I react to that with childish defiance. (P2)

I clear up the situation at work. I've taken sick leave until the end of my probationary period and sent in my notice directly after. (P2)

Developing more of an interest in energy work. (P4)

Doubts, decision-making, fear of decisions

Now I've got doubts again and trouble making decisions. Can I actually manage this or did I take on too much? Do I have the nerves for it? (P2)

Vulnerable/unprotected

My colleague's desolate condition saps my strength, her depression pulls me down somewhat. (P1)

Invulnerable/protection

I feel invulnerable, as if I had the proverbial thick skin or some kind of strong shell that surrounds me like a protective shield. However, it feels as if the protection comes from within, not as if I have some kind of shield put over top of me. It feels really, really good. At the beginning of the proving (I was) strong, positive, calm with myself, yet disconnected from the world at large, but in a good way. Nothing could hurt or destroy me. It was like I was surrounded by a shield. It felt like a shine from within. (P1)

My fears have flipped to absolute calm. Like: "It'll work out in the end". (P3)

Positive feeling of "Bite me!", I feel more resistant. (P4)

Spiritually good, slight feeling of being above things, or rather, not only the others are important, I am too. (P5)

Happiness and satisfaction because I was able to help my uncle. (P5)

Since taking the remedy I am generally braver. I don't get worked up so much over things I cannot change. I'm no longer so "tactful" to people who are not tactful to me. (P5)

People (taxi drivers, neighbors, colleagues) are suddenly even more open and trusting of me. I am less afraid. (P5)

Separated, excluded, lost contact, old

I have the feeling like I've fallen into a hole. I feel old, lonesome, ugly, excluded, separated from the world and other people. It's like I've lost contact. (P1)

Now I've finished inside myself too, but feel more lost inside me for it. The outside is dark and far away. Inside, there is still life, but without connection. The light no longer reaches outside. (P1)

I try for loving empathy and attention, but I feel that I cannot relate. It's like I'm light years away from the topic (wish for child), indifferent and disconnected. (P1)

In regards to relationships and interaction with other people I feel completely disconnected in my current state, in my little capsule (light inside, but muted), surrounded by impassable blackness (dark outside), as if I would never again come into contact and communication with others. (P1)

Feeling depressed. The depression shows me: you're already old. Who would still want you? Have no illusions? (P2)

I just wasn't in my head. I felt like in a fog the entire day. Suddenly, the veil was lifted and I was able to laugh again. (P2)

Retreat, breaking contact to protect self

Several times, I've seriously thought about breaking off contact, because it gets me so down, seeing that toxic relationship and the pain that they always renew and deepen. (P1)

Contact to an old acquaintance that interpreted our relationship as more than it was. All I can say about that is: "Kiss my ass!". I'm always nice to everyone and I'm happy when we can laugh together. That this attitude gets turned on me like some kind of love story I really can't tolerate. I told him right to his face, that I won't in a million years reciprocate anything of what he's interpreting. It gets me really angry that they always think that way and ruin a fun friendship. (P2)

Many people approach me, making me think: "What do they all even want from me?" (P2)

I have little wish for masses of people. I stayed at home all day. (P3)

Calm and balance

I feel good. It's a relaxed day. (P1)

I feel in balance and in a positive mood. (P1)

Did relaxing Yoga with my daughter and watched kids' films. (P1)

The remainder of the day and evening goes nicely and without any special happenings. (P1)

Relaxation during a cosmetic treatment: many incidental memories surface. Short images of my mother-in-law, an inter-section in America (where we used to live), short scenes, my grandparents' home village. All of it nice and peaceful, loving and cheerful, like home. (P1)

The days go calmly, harmonically and without noteworthy events. (P1)

I keep on. There comes a healing. I am calm, braced. (P2)

Confident, positive, calm, stressless. (P4)

Could be that I'm more self-confident. (P4)

Good mood, confidence, no more fear from news etc., slightly "rebellious", telling my mind. (P5)

Calm, even in the face of oncoming stress, "I have to keep my thoughts together", but feel strength nonetheless. (P5)

Sadness

Sadness because of an argument: in my current state it saddens me deeply. I feel like people just aren't made to live together in harmony. (P1)

Sadness because of the current geopolitical situation. (P1)

I feel no more laughter in me. (P1)

It feels like there is still a sob in my chest that could break back out at any moment. (P1)

Slightly melancholy in relation to menstruation, but my mood improves together with my bodily condition. (P5)

Indifference, demotivation

This week the overarching theme was: "Nothing is important to me anymore!" (P2)

Irritability

I am very tired and pretty irritable in the evenings. (P1)

I'm irritable, also toward other adults. ... said to me, I should laugh again sometime. (P2)

Overcoming something together, motivation

Yoga with friends: now, several of these online girl friends had the same motivation and together it works really wonderfully! Daily, we exchange our experiences with the lesson of the day and motivate each other. (P1)

Actually, I was feeling dead tired and unmotivated. To my great joy, the program went super well today and was a lot of fun. I feel energized and balanced. (P1)

Powerful, energetic

Despite my headache, I feel otherwise good and in a positive mood. (P1)

Despite not taking any breaks, I am full of power and can handle and finish everything. (P1)

The way it's going right now is good as it is. I am so full of power; I've got a positive feeling and a great energy inside of me. (P2)

The last couple of days, I've been following through more, I've finished things I started and beat my own laziness better. (P3)

I've done thing right away. (P3)

Empathetic yet still free

At the same time, I am able to get in the same vibe as others and their emotions, without adopting them for myself. I notice how I'm especially able to be present and empathetic in difficult situations (a girl friend's love problems; controversies etc.) without putting my own feeling in the foreground. I take nothing personally. I feel free. (P1)

Empathy affects negatively

Concerning his story, however, I suffer with him especially, I feel (his) great sadness and within myself a great anger at his and his wife's unwillingness and inability to get to an arrangement or end the relationship. (P1)

Grief with lack of drive

Death of a neighbor and childhood friend, the tragic circumstances and the fact that he was the first from my childhood generation to die an unwanted death, really threw me off track.

The burial was on 02/08/2017. Since then, I've been feeling smashed. The days after I could hardly work, not think clearly, as if I had a hangover. (I'm normally very resilient and seldom get big mood swings, especially not grief. Normally, I would experience grief in combination with gratefulness or happiness over shared experiences.) (P1)

Appointments, procrastination, forgetfulness

All the time, I'm very forgetful, especially where it concerns important dates. I have to take them down into my phone. (P2)

Postponing appointments for personal talks all the time, then I forget them. (P3)

It is generally difficult to remember appointments. But it has now become somewhat better. (P3)

Unease, crowded thoughts, "can I handle everything?",
I'm stressed, under time pressure, have lots of appointments and/or deadlines. (P5)

Travel

Managed a long journey well. (P4)

Recurring dream: I go travelling and have too much luggage with me. (P5)

An upcoming journey is stressing me out, but already better on the way back and when I was home after travelling. (P5)

Unfulfilled wish for child

My best friend wants to have a third child and cannot get pregnant because of health problems. She's really suffering and is now even going to visit a planned parenthood clinic. (P1)

Marriage crisis, separation

My best male friend is (once again) in an ugly marriage crisis. His marriage has been a catastrophe from the beginning, but he is unable and unwilling to go through with divorce. (P1)

Dreams

Dream with my mother. An argument. Suddenly, my whole body is covered in large pustules, one next to the next. My mother is yelling at somebody: "Look, see how she looks now!". After that, more arguing and yelling with tears. (I don't know any more detail; I often have argumentative dreams with my mother) (P1)

A family get-together with my uncle's entire family. We live in a very large house. All the furnishing is very high-class, but also comfortable and homey; many sofas, armchairs, blankets and cushions. The entire bottom floor is an enormous living room, occupied by the entire extended family. The mood is calm and pleasant. Everybody's occupied, playing games or making conversation.

I have to go number 2 and find that the toilets are on the edge of this giant room. It is built into a long couch. I have a seat on this sofa and find it very unpleasant that I'm supposed to do my business in the giant room, among all my relations.

My cousin's wife comes and sits, newspaper in hand, on the other end of the toilet sofa. I ask her, if she has to go as well. She denies this and says that she simply wanted to retreat a bit. She says she needs this every day, just being able to retreat for two hours. She uses this time to read the paper.

I point out, that this is the toilet sofa and I really have to go and ask her to please go somewhere else. She simply refuses this, gets comfortable on the sofa, puts her feet up and begins reading the news.

I am upset at this and feel misunderstood. I leave the house in anger and march up the street. There are other houses, but I feel a bit lost. Several members of my family are following me and want to mediate, but I am inconsolable and the cousin is still being unreasonable. (P1)

Many dreams, but not memorable. (P1)

People that are searching for something or have to complete some tasks and somehow, I'm involved. Either I'm helping out or I need to solve some problem myself. (P1)

One of the dreams was kind of like that, but I was somehow "trapped". A man had me under control in a room (no violence) and I just couldn't leave, instead I dreamed up possible ways out of the situation in my sleep. (P1)

At night, I had another dream in which many people from my life appeared, people I'm no longer in contact with. (P1)

This dream again occurs in a large house, where everybody lives together. This time, there are lots of (bed)rooms surrounding a large living room. All attending are there with their partners. Several of these friends/acquaintances (there were no relatives) are trying to convince me that I, too, need a partner and how important a relationship is. They're all so proud of their partners and relationships.

This quite alienates me. I have no inclination to start a relationship and all this talk of "but you have to!" really gets on my nerves. I know that one of my exes is waiting in the first room. However, I really don't understand why I should go (back) into that room with him. (At the beginning of the dream, I had left his room to be in the living room). Except for something sexual, I haven't the slightest interest in getting together with this person, however I know that I won't be able to avoid the whole package if I go back into that room. So, I stay in the living room, which action is met with nonunderstanding from the rest of the community. But I don't care. I feel totally satisfied and in harmony with myself. (P1)

I know that I had a dream where a man was trying to establish contact to my child. I know that he wants to abuse my child (I can't remember whether it was my actual daughter or whether I had a different child here). I must prevent him from realizing his plan. I must not be outsmarted or tricked by him. He is very skillful and eloquent, but as long as I stand between him and my child, nothing can happen. I have to watch out, so he can't pull a quick move and get past me. It's like a game of mental strength and skill. (P1)

My dreams at night are still very varied and intense. At the moment, they have this quality of failure and trying in vain. (P1)

I have dreams of disappointing people. They try hard to show me something beautiful and I don't react correctly. I can feel their disappointment, their anger. I get the feeling "I'm not doing it right". (P1)

In other dreams, they're trying to trick me. They make it clear to me that I don't belong. I am presented a situation and consequently told that I'm not wanted there. (P1)

I had a dream where they were taking semen from stallions, to effect artificial inseminations. First, the horses had to be made to urinate. I remember immense quantities of urine from the horses. The semen collection itself I cannot remember. I was a watcher in the dream, an amateur visitor and wondered about the methods. But I dared not ask questions, because as a non-professional I obviously had no idea, so I didn't belong there. At the same time, the dream had some kind of sexual quality. This is definitely remarkable, as it's the only time in a dream of mine where animals and sexuality have ever occurred in connection, even in the context of a remedy test. (P1)

I'm dreaming again, with and about Katharina (great grand-mother). All the time during the last 3 weeks since the beginning of this proving I haven't had any dreams. (P2)

Dream about a carnival. I had a costume on, some kind of clown. People were laughing at me, because it looked so ugly. I had green frizzy hair. I woke up during the laughter. (P2)

Dreams of getting together with a man, not being alone. (P2)

Dreams of one of my sons. He's begun an apprenticeship as a barber. He'd grown tall, and was cutting like Edward Scissorhands, that was great. He was looking posh, very neat. (P2)

Recurring dream: I go on a journey and have too much luggage. (P5)

Terrible dreams: for example, I see a meteor hitting earth and I take my family, who are sitting around the table with me, by the hands. Everybody's smiling, then comes the tremor. (P5)

I had a dream that I killed two people. I made them disappear. The dream felt so real that I wasn't sure whether it actually was a dream after waking up. (P5)

Head

I just wasn't in my right mind. I felt like I was in a fog the whole day. (P2)

Things were happening more and more in the brain. It was like a movement in the brain, it was positive, as if the brain was being stretched, like brain gymnastics. (P3)

Head, headache

Since about noon, I've had a headache in the front vertex. It's a pulse that also causes a pulsing pressure in the base of the nose. (P1)

On the first day of my period, I had a relatively strong headache, right side, under the crown. (P1)

Headache accompanied by diarrhea. Went away quickly, though. (P3)

Repeatedly got light headaches, pressing (more often than usual). (P5)

Head, facial swelling

It feels like my face is swollen, puffy, as if I had cried for days on end. (P1)

Swollen lower right eyelid. It seems extremely pronounced again for the past three weeks. It feels swollen, more than you can see in the mirror. (P1)

Eye, lachrymation

For a few days, I had a runny eye (right side), especially in the mornings. The flow of tears was mild, but I had to keep dabbing it throughout the day, because it simply wouldn't stop. (P1)

Heart

Falling asleep difficult because of heart palpitations, at night, <when lying on back, blubbering in the heart with a feeling as though something is blocked; > getting up, < laying down.

More seldom during the day, < in the evening when sitting on the couch, blubbering feeling and the light feeling of blockage. (From about 20:30) (P1)

Abdomen, flatulence/pinching

A totally bloated belly in the evening (after 19:00) that goes down putridly on the toilet. (P1)

Putrid flatulence, smell is repulsively manure- and rot-like, without abdominal bloating. (P1)

Pinching in the belly – feeling of fighting off infection. (P4)

Abdomen, pain right side, stomach pain

In my lower right abdomen, I can sometimes feel a soft swelling. The pain is often like a side stitch, so that I feel short of breath, despite not having moved. This pain often radiates out toward the liver, seldom toward the back (about the kidney area). (P1)

Otherwise, I had a lot of body pains over the last week; mostly in the upper abdomen and more on the right side, < bread, bread rolls. (P1)

After eating a bread roll, after about half an hour to an hour, cramping pain in the upper abdomen, lasting for about an hour. (P1)

Pinching in the belly. (P4)

Feeling like a stone in the stomach after drinking red wine with a high acidity. (P4)

Back

Slight pain in lower back, like previously, lumbar spine, pressing, enduring < when lying down, sitting, standing, came out of nowhere. (P5)

Extremities, looseness, relaxation, need to move

Very loosely swinging arms after workout. (P4)

My calves feel extremely loose, I have an urge to move. (P4)

Pain, hip

I got up and my left hip is hurting. It feels like a contusion, but I can't see anything. < cold and touching, clothes contact, > warmth, lying on it, during sleep. (P2)

The hip pain is really only noticeable in the morning and evening. During the day there's a lot going on, than I don't feel anything and don't even think about it. (P2)

Pulling in groin, complaint old rupture

Had an operation a few years ago because of an inguinal hernia on both sides. I used to have intermittent problems, a pulling pain < intensive play of football/soccer. But now, after these four weeks, that's super too. (P3)

Pulling pain in right groin, more specifically in the transition between leg and pelvis, as if the leg wasn't on properly < in movement, > at rest, (was only around for a day). (P5)

Pain knee

Before the proving, problems in the knee pit, can't get up from a squat, pain pulls to the rear. At the end of the proving, my knee problems have all but gone. No more pain. (P3)

Feedback six weeks after first intake: knee problems have completely disappeared, no more problems despite intensively playing football/soccer. (P3)

Sore muscles in upper arms

Feeling of muscle ache in upper arms, only noticeable during movement. (P5)

Menstruation

I had relatively strong pains in the lower right abdominal area, that I found impairing. The pain radiated into the entire right abdomen. (P1)

On the first day of my period, I had a relatively strong headache, right side, under the crown. (P1)

My menses had normalized so nicely over the past couple of months. Now, everything is back to how it was before. I'm in pain and irritable. The discharge is stronger again and so is the smell. (P2)

My PMS ailments (chest tightness, water retention, bad mood, pain in lower back, endless appetite) disappeared right after taking the first globules. (P5)

Temperature

I get very cold < in the evening. (P5)

Freezing, > in the sun, warmth. (P5)

Sweat

I'm sweating a lot at night during sleep from the torso, so much so that my top and the blanket get moist. (P1)

I sweat very strongly. (P2)

I break out in sweats at night, so bad! (P3)

Attack of sweating at 3 AM. (P3)

Attacks of sweating at night (often in connections to the bad dreams). (P5)

Alternately sweating and freezing during sleep, the sweating feels feverish. (P5)

Skin, hair

Hair is very beautiful, it's lustrous and growing especially quickly at the moment, same thing with my nails. (P2)

Breakouts on the head, pimples or rather like subterranean pimples, elevations in the skin, not itchy. (P3)

Pimples in face, like acne, but gone again after three days. (P3)

Vertigo

During sauna work I wasn't feeling well, got dizzy. (P2)

From 20:00 massive circulation problems, < sitting, walking; > laying down in bed; dizzy as if I was drunk, back and forth like a carnival swing; afraid I'd keel over. (P3)

Several times had circulation problems with dizziness. (P3)

Injuries

Fell badly during soccer on Sunday. The left arm was contused and like dislocated. I took some pain medication, because the arm hurt so badly. But I was surprised to see that the next day, there was only a little swelling left, but the arm was already fully mobile again. Incredibly fast healing. I know these kinds of injuries; they normally take much longer. (P3)

Had an operation a few years ago because of an inguinal hernia on both sides. I used to have intermittent problems. But now, after these four weeks, that's super too. (P3)

Sleep

Falling asleep difficult because of heart palpitations, at night < lying on back. (P1)

Wake up at night, 2 AM, difficult to fall back asleep, very unusual for me. (P4)

Bad sleep, wake up every hour. (P5)

Don't sleep so well < full moon. (P5)

General

Improved defense from infections, very robust health, despite wife and child being ill. (P4)

Throat pain from first day of taking remedy, different than usual, got deeper voice, < speaking, > drinking. (P5)

Case studies

Cases from my own practice

Female, 20, recurring tendinitis, fears

She's been having wrist problems for a few years. Ten years ago, her wrist was terribly swollen. Four years later, a ganglion was diagnosed and operated on. This happened again twice over the course of the next four years, first on the right side, then on the left. She was operated on each time.

Acutely, she has tendinitis in the right wrist. The wrist is swollen from time to time. She gets sudden strong pains she describes as pressing and pulsating. Rest >, movement <.

This is already the third inflammation within the past year. So far, treatment has consisted of Ibuprofen, 600 mg tablets.

Furthermore, she sometime gets headaches. These are pulsating and pressing, > by lying down, < from noise.

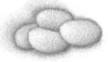

That then feels as if someone was stomping around on her head. Standing <. Too little sleep and stress at work are possible triggers.

Her back also causes her difficulties. For example, her back is crooked, the right shoulder pulls up too far, a vertebra is displaced in her cervical spine and her lumbar spine locks up. She gets a stabbing pain in the solar plexus area, as if someone jabbed something in there. This sometimes gets so bad that she doubles over, < sitting down, > breathing normally and taking deep breaths.

She doesn't currently know where she's going. That's her greatest challenge at the moment, not knowing where her life is supposed to go.

As a person, she describes herself as timid. She worries a lot about her family and relatives, is afraid something might happen to them. She's also afraid of not being able to help. She's still very sad about her grandmother's death (nine years ago) and her cousin's. The cousin died of cancer and since then, she's been afraid of cancer as well.

Her three greatest wishes are to get her grandma and cousin back and never having to hear about cancer ever again.

Prescription: *Sericum coconum LMXM*, 2x daily

Follow-up consultation six weeks later:
The inflammation is much improved, no more headaches, nor more backaches, her fears have ameliorated. Emotionally, she feels much more relaxed and confident.

However, she now has more stress at work. She's taken on a second job and drinks a lot of coffee now, has heartburn a lot more often > lemon water.

Prescription: *Sericum coconum LMXM* as before, until the wrist is completely alright, additionally *Nux vomica LM12* for acute heartburn.

Feedback half a year later
She's doing very well. So far, no more problems with the wrists. Neither the back- nor headaches have returned. She's noticed that she has to change her diet, as the heartburn is obviously connected to the increased consumption of coffee.

She got some advice about correcting her diet depending on her breathing type and adjusted her diet accordingly.

Since then, no further treatment has been necessary.

Female, 45, fear of upcoming air travel

The woman is supposed to travel by air to a somewhat remote region of India for business purposes. She's accompanying a guide dog from her own school that an Indian woman had her train. This is a great adventure for her, because there are several hurdles to overcome here. Therefore, she is very afraid that something might go wrong on the journey, that either she or the dog might not arrive at their destination in one piece. Because of this, she hasn't been able to sleep properly for a good while and is, on the whole, very anxious and unsettled.

Prescription: *Sericum coconum C200,* once a week until the start of travel and then three times on the day of departure. If need be, she can repeat the ingestion in India.

Feedback from the patient after the journey

It was totally relaxed. I instantly noticed that I could sleep better and got more confident.

The journey itself went very well, despite having some problems I hadn't anticipated. I was able to handle everything calmly and well. I gave the remedy to the dog as well, who was also very anxious and calmed down a lot from it.

Male, 48, recurring tendon injuries, induration palm

His clinical history of the past few years consists of recurring injuries of tendons and ligaments several times a year. Bicep's tendon rupture in the right while warming up for sports, torn ligament in left foot (several times). Currently has a left side shoulder injury that makes it difficult for him to move his arm forward. This injury occurred from overexertion while remodeling an apartment. One doctor diagnosed him with ruptured cartilage, another with arthritis. He self-medicated with *Ruta graveolens C200*, without amelioration however.

He is an athletic type with a high desire for exercise, who has trouble knowing and remembering his limits in sports. For this reason, he has previously taken *Arnica montana* and *Rhus toxicodendron*. In the case of this acute injury, I also first prescribed him *Arnica montana*, followed by *Rhus toxicodendron*. This however did not yield the intended result, so that I followed it up with *Sericum coconum* in alternation with *Rhus toxicodendron* in increasing LM potencies over the course of three months.

My choice of *Sericum coconum* was further strengthened by his fear of flying, with an especial phobia of crashing. This, too, improved remarkably after taking the remedy.

Another positive change occurred with his skin. The skin on his torso was always very sensitive to synthetic fibers such as polyester. Upon contact, it would start to itch and sting, which got even worse when sweating. During treatment, this improved quite a bit.

Last contact was a year after treatment. So far, he hadn't had anymore injuries. The induration of the tendons in his hands had become much better. He did not wish to be further treated for this. He also tells me that some positive changes have occurred in his life. He now has an easier time adjusting to changes (work/private life).

Female, 46, stretched ligament right ankle

Right foot, outside, by tripping down stairs, bad pain, strong swelling and hypermobility of joint, symptoms ameliorate almost suddenly after taking *Sericum coconum C10,000*.
Within 12 hours the pain and swelling have disappeared, which had previously been unsuccessfully treated with *Arnica montana*, *Ruta graveolens* and *Bellis perennis*. Within a week, normal mobility of the joint has been restored. Despite having this kind of accident quite often in the past, it has not reoccurred since taking *Sericum coconum*. (Observed over a span of 10 years).

Female, 68, stretched ligament right ankle

Right foot, outside, from rolling her ankle while walking on even ground, treated with *Sericum coconum C200* and *C10,000*. According to her attending physician, the injury healed astonishingly quickly for a woman of her age. After about four weeks, the patient was able to walk without a support bandage. Pain and swelling were already completely gone after roughly two weeks.

Girl, 11, partially torn LCL of ankle joint

Partially torn LCL of the right ankle from rolling the joint during jumping exercises in PE at school, prescribed *Sericum coconum C200*, dissolved in water several times a day when in pain, very fast healing within two weeks.

Male, 48, lumbar disk herniation with inflammation

He works as a courier driver, meaning he is on the go all day, as well as carrying heavy things a lot. Despite this, he enjoys his job. He really wants to go back to work as a courier, which is currently impossible due to strong pain in the back L3/L4, pressing, pulling, radiating into the legs. Diagnosis: disc prolapse. Furthermore, his right foot is without sensation. The inactivity is really getting to him. He cannot sit still, despite the movement making his pain a lot worse.

The first acute treatment was *Arnica montana* and *Hypericum C10,000*, with no significant improvement. Because his physician additionally diagnosed an inflammation in the area of his prolapse, I decide on *Sericum coconum C10,000*, once every second day.

This leads to an improvement and after three weeks he is almost free from pain.

Sadly, he is very impatient. He uses his relative painlessness to quickly go back to work as a courier. After three weeks on the job, the symptoms reoccur. He is treated once again with *Sericum coconum C10,000*, this time in alternation with *Hypericum C10,000*.

With this treatment for three weeks, he is painless for over half a year. However, soon after going back to work as a courier, he suffers another disc prolapse. Since he doesn't want to give up his work as a courier, his physician recommends an operation on his spine, which he goes through with. Since then, he isn't being treated by me anymore.

A year later, he tells me that the pain has come back despite the operation and that he finally decided to give up his occupation and take another job.

Male cat, 6 months, stretched ligament right hind leg

The young tomcat got his hind leg caught while jumping and injured it in the process. He was unable to move it and it jutted unnaturally outward. An X-Ray at the veterinarian showed a stretched ligament (possibly torn, but this would have required further scans at a specialist). The bones were all fine.

He was treated with *Sericum coconum C10,000*, three times on the first day, once a day thereafter. He consequently started walking again, initially only a few steps to his litter box or food bowl. After about a week he was once again able to walk normally, albeit slowly and cautiously. After about a month he was again fit enough to spend time with the other cat and run around some. He took a lot longer to start jumping again, however.

In the four years that have passed since the accident, he would occasionally start limping again. Giving him *Sericum coconum C200* usually helped quickly.

Male, 59, groin strain through rotation while lifting, report on self-treatment

I was lifting a suitcase from my car, shortly after there came a stabbing pain in the right groin, radiating toward the abdomen. At first, I thought it was the appendix, judging from the pain. I used to have an irritated appendix from time to time, but changing my diet accordingly brought no improvement. The pain was a bit worse in movement. Turning over in bed was especially painful, so there wasn't really an improvement at night.

I then took *Arnica montana C10,000*. That didn't help, neither did *Rhus toxicodendron C200*. Then, I thought of the *Sericum coconum C10,000* which I'd been taking a while ago for another injury. After the first intake I noticed an improvement right away. I took it three times the first day. This caused the stabbing groin pain to recede. Two days later, it was completely gone.

Sericum coconum in family planning treatment

In my practice, I often start treatment for women wishing to get pregnant with *Sericum coconum*. It helps these women to clearly and explicitly decide on their way to their child, removes doubts and fears and thereby, gives them surety on their further path. This is especially important where many different methods have already been employed to no avail and the woman/the couple is unsure if it can even "still work", about getting a child.

The following is an account of a patient of mine after three quarters of a year of treatment. She had already had several miscarriages and unsuccessfully tried in vitro fertilization several times. During homeopathic treatment, spontaneous fertilization occurred for the first time. Sadly, she was unable to carry this child to term as well. However, she's keeping on with her homeopathic treatment with confidence in the future and in herself. Quote: "I'm very confident and once again trust in myself and my strengths and I've gotten back into harmony with myself again."

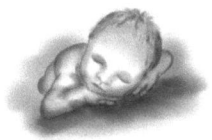

Sericum coconum as a protective remedy

Sericum coconum has proven an effective remedy when a deep development process takes place during treatment, when a patient feels unprotected and vulnerable. They wish for inner strength to better isolate themselves from other people.

I like to give it to them as an acute remedy ahead of difficult challenges. It also works well when taking as an intermediate remedy. The patient is able to gain calm, confidence and strength for the treatment to come, especially when it comes to mental illnesses.

Cases from homeopath Renate Siefert

Own experiences concerning travel

Shortly after triturating silk and producing a C30 myself, I travelled by airplane. Usually, I'm quite anxious ahead of flying and uptight during flight. With "*Silk C30*", three times five globules the day before and the day of, I was really able to enjoy the flight; it was great to be in the air and to see the world from above.

Male, 57, chronic tendinitis of the Achilles tendon and afflictions from travel

This man was practically born on skis. In his home in Norway, he was athletically active from childhood: skiing in the winter, mountain climbing in the summer. He's a nervous, unsettled type of person. When he comes to me for treatment, he's 52 years old and has been suffering from tendinitis of the Achilles tendon for ten years. His symptoms get better or worse depending on physical strain. We begin his treatment in March 2012. After ski season, his affliction is very pronounced; he can only walk with a limp, his lower leg is painful.

I prescribe him *Sericum coconum C1,000*, five globules to be taken once a week. Within the next four weeks, the pain gets better, after eight weeks he's showing no more symptoms.

After mountaineering season, in September 2012, he once again complains of pain. Once again, I prescribe *Sericum coconum C1,000*, five globules to be taken once a week. He gets better, after three weeks there are no more complaints.

At the beginning of December, I asked him to return before skiing season, so that we can absorb some of the coming physical strain with medication.

Just by the by, he mentions having to travel a lot for work now. This, he says, stresses him out quite a bit, as he just doesn't like being on the go all the time.

I gave him 5 globules of *Sericum coconum C1,000* during the consultation and once again prescribed him to take the C1,000 weekly until February.

In March 2013, he came back to me for a shoulder injury. His Achilles tendon hadn't caused any more grief, despite the physical strain from skiing. When I asked him about the stress from the constant travel, he answered that he had almost no trouble with that anymore; on the contrary, he was enjoying it now, travelling and seeing a lot. Now, he saw lots of positives in all the travel. (Complaints from travel had indeed shown themselves to be a key note with *Sericum coconum*.)

I gave him a tube of *Sericum coconum C200* for his travel first-aid kit and recommended he occasionally take five globules in case of physical strain or exceeding stress on journeys. Now and again, we meet. He has no more complaints.

Female, physiotherapist, 52, chronic tendinitis in both forearms/wrists

She has been my patient for years because of other unrelated complaints. Now, she laments strong pains in both wrists, radiating to the forearms, stemming from work stress as a physio-therapist.

During consultation, I give her five globules *Sericum coconum C10,000* and prescribe that she takes another five per week, for a total of six weeks. After that, she was free of complaints. As a prophylactic, she takes five globules of *Sericum coconum C200* ahead of exceptional workloads. She's enthusiastic about this new homeopathic remedy.

Feedback from homeopath Anne Schadde

I've used silk *(Sericum coconum)* several times now. Specifically, when ailments of tendons and ligaments are indicated.

Patient 1: A cruciate ligament rupture showed a connection again, despite it being very unusual for a complete rupture to heal up.

Patient 2: Two years after an operation on her cruciate ligament, she got such strong pain, that she had to go to hospital on crutches. Nobody was able to explain what had happened. By taking Silk (*Sericum coconum*) she was able to walk and bend the knee again after a few days.

Patient 3: Partial LCL rupture, after two days already showing a reorganization of the entire foot.

Mother reports on her child's treatment
Boy 11, frequent rolling of ankles

His most recent injury was quite severe, so a visit to the doctor was in order.

Our experience with *Sericum coconum C200* is a very positive one. Up until the second checkup, everything indicated a ruptured ligament, or at least a partial rupture, or possibly even a broken bone at the enthesis and my son wasn't allowed to put any weight on the foot at all.

The second checkup two weeks later – which was about a week after taking the remedy – revealed, after an X-Ray, that the foot is in good shape and that there's no problem with the ligaments or tendons, only the epiphyseal plate is somewhat stretched.

Meaning: he's allowed to put a load on the foot again and in two weeks he can carefully take up sports again. Amazingly enough, the doctor then claimed that children of his age (11 years) almost never rupture ligaments, because they're still so stable. I took that with some skepticism.

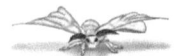

Homeopathic remedy picture of Sericum coconum bombyx mori (ser-coc)

Sign
Untreated silk cocoon of the domestic silk moth Bombyx mori, origin China

Affinity
Mind, tendons, ligaments, cartilage, skin, hair, women.

Modalities
Worse: before and during travel, life changes, motion
Better: rest, after finishing travel, fresh air.

Key symptoms
Injuries of tendons and ligaments.
Travel ailments.
Lack of protection.
Skin/hair problems.

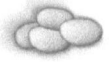

Main themes and symptoms

Mind

M   Fear of making choices (1)(3)(5)

M   Departure/vigor/motivation – lack of drive (1)(5)

M   Divided/left out/retreat – sociable (5)

M   Inner strength, assertiveness (1)(5)

M   Travel (1)(2)(4)(5)
- Fear of travel, with anxiety
- Disturbed sleep ahead of travel
- Dislike of/stress from travel
- Fear of flying
- Fear that something might happen en route
- Fear of not arriving at destination

M   Calm and poise – irritability (1)(5)

M   Protection/invulnerability – unprotected/vulnerable (3)(5)

M   Forgetfulness, appointments (5)

M   Desire to wear silk clothing (1)(3)

M   Confidence and happiness – sadness (1)(5)

General

G   Sleep, restful (3)

G   Perspiration, ample, at night (5)

G   Sunlight, sun heat agg. (1)

G   Dreams (1)(3)(6)
- About travel
- Trouble on journeys
- Too much baggage on journeys
- Catastrophes
- Family, family arguments
- Looking strange, being mocked for it

Physical

P   **Headaches (5)**
- Right side under the crown during menstruation
- Pulsing pressure under front vertex
- Headaches accompanied by diarrhea
- Slight headaches, pressing

P   **Skin and hair (1)(3)(5)**

P   **Back, disc prolapse (2)**

P   **Back, pain, pressing (2)(5)**

P   **Extremities, tendons and ligaments (1)(2)(4)(5)(6)**
- Sprained and ruptured ligament, ankle
- Tendinitis in wrist, lower arms, both sides
- Tendinitis in Achilles tendon
- Sprained and ruptured LCL
- Ruptured ACL

P   **Frequent rolling of ankle (1)(2)(6)**

P   Female reproductive organs (5)
- Strong pains, lower right abdomen, radiating into entire abdomen
- Menstruation accompanied by headache
- PMS (irritability, pressure in chest, wateriness, back ache, endless appetite)
- Discharge, foul smelling

(1)   Notes after intake of Silk C10,000, 2005
(2)   Patient cases from practice Katrin Rabe, 2007-2020
(3)   C4 trituration and experiences with self-made C4, 2008
(4)   Feedback from homeopath Renate Siefert, 2008-2019
(5)   Proving 2016-2017
(6)   Further feedback

Remedy comparisons

In my own practice, I have noted similarities between the remedy *Sericum coconum* and the following other remedies, sorted by key symptoms:

Injuries and inflammation of tendons and ligaments
- *Anacardium:* lack of decisiveness, difficulty of making choices, injury of tendons, more Achilles tendon.
- *Ruta graveolens*: the injury/inflammation of tendons was often the result of overexertion without the specific problem of "finding one's way".

Ailments related to travel
- *Cocculus, Petroleum, Tabacum, Nux vomica:* Car sickness
- *Calcium phosphoricum:* Desire to travel and, when under-way, desire to go back home.
- *Aconitum:* Fear of flying, then often in conjunction with panic attacks, tachycardia and/or shortness of breath.

Lack of protection

- *Vernix caseosa*: Feeling of lacking protection, mental vulnerability with sensitivity to external influences like noise, improved by holding ears shut.
- *Astacus fluviatilis*: Feeling of lacking a protective layer; feeling of being too soft; quote from patient: "I'd like to have armor around me, to defend from enemy attacks from the outside, so I can finish my development in peace."
- *Hermit crabs* (e.g. deep sea hermit crabs Parapaguridae): Feel vulnerable and exposed, want to retreat to a house/room; quote from patient: "I'd like to have a house I could carry with me at all times, so that I could hop into it if need be."

Hair/skin

- *Tela aranea:* dry, itchy skin – with *Tela aranea* (spider's web) the itch was accompanied by the feeling as if a web was spreading over the body, starting from the crotch; there was also a visible nettle-like rash. With *Sericum coconum*, this rash is less pronounced.
- *Silicea:* a good follow-up to Silk, inner strength, skin
- *Sulphur:* itchy skin, wool agg.

The following remedies might also be considered

- Byssus silk of the fan mussel *Pinna nobilis*: because of a similar make-up and emergence of the substance.
- Butterflies e. g. *Bombyx mori:* because butterfly remedies support development processes, often seem delicate and vulnerable.

Follows well on: *Arnica montana, Bellis perennis,*
                                   Ruta graveolens
Complementary to: *Symphytum, Arnica montana,*
                                   Ruta graveolens

Repertory

I suggest that the following symptoms are adopted into the repertories.

- MIND - ANXIETY - journey; before a
- MIND - ANXIETY - travelling; before
- MIND - ANXIETY - future, about
- MIND - AILMENTS FROM - anticipation
- MIND - CARES, full of - future; about
- MIND - CHILDREN - beget and to have children; desire to
- MIND - FEAR - flying; of - airplane; in
- MIND - FEAR - travelling, of
- MIND - IRRITABILITY - menses - before
- MIND - MENSES - before
- MIND - THOUGHTS - future, of the
- MIND - TRAVELLING - desire for

- VERTIGO - VERTIGO

- HEAD - HAIR - brittle
- HEAD - HAIR - dryness
- HEAD - PAIN - extending to - Nose - Root of nose - pulsating pain

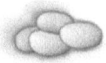

- HEAD - PAIN - lying - amel. - pressing pain
- HEAD - PAIN - menses - during - agg. - pressing pain
- HEAD - PAIN - noise - agg.
- HEAD - PAIN - pressing pain
- HEAD - PAIN - pulsating pain
- HEAD - PAIN - standing - agg. - pressing pain

- EYE - PHOTOPHOBIA - light; from - sunlight - agg.

- STOMACH - NAUSEA - airplane; in an
- STOMACH - NAUSEA - riding - bus; on a - agg.
- STOMACH - NAUSEA - riding - carriage; in a - agg.

- BACK - INFLAMMATION - Joints - accompanied by - herniated disk
- BACK - PAIN - motion - agg.
- BACK - PAIN - turning - agg.
- BACK - PAIN - turning - agg. - drawing pain
- BACK - PAIN - Lumbar region - motion - agg. - pressing pain
- BACK - PAIN - Lumbar region - motion - agg. - sudden motion - aching
- BACK - PAIN - Lumbar region - motion - agg. - drawing pain

- BACK - PAIN - Lumbar region - turning - agg. - suddenly - aching
- BACK - PAIN - Lumbar region - turning - body - agg. - drawing pain
- BACK - PAIN - Lumbar region - extending to - Legs - drawing pain
- BACK - PAIN - Lumbar region - rest - amel. - pressing pain
- BACK - PAIN - Lumbar region - sitting - agg. - pressing pain
- BACK - PROLAPSUS - Intervertebral disk

- EXTREMITIES - DISLOCATION; EASY - Ankles
- EXTREMITIES - DISLOCATION - Ankles
- EXTREMITIES - GIVE WAY - Ankles
- EXTREMITIES - GANGLION - Wrist, on
- EXTREMITIES - INFLAMMATION - Wrists
- EXTREMITIES - INFLAMMATION - Tendons
- EXTREMITIES - INFLAMMATION - Legs - Tendo Achillis
- EXTREMITIES - INJURIES - Tendons
- EXTREMITIES - INJURIES - Legs - Tendo Achillis
- EXTREMITIES - PAIN - Wrists
- EXTREMITIES - PAIN - Wrists - twisting agg.
- EXTREMITIES - PAIN - Upper arms - Biceps
- EXTREMITIES - PAIN - Legs - Tendo Achillis

- EXTREMITIES - RUPTURE of ligaments - Legs - Tendo Achillis
- EXTREMITIES - SPRAINS - Wrists
- EXTREMITIES - SPRAINS - Ankles
- EXTREMITIES - SPRAINS - Ankles - right
- EXTREMITIES - SPRAINS - Ankles - recurrent
- EXTREMITIES - UNSTEADINESS, joints - Feet
- EXTREMITIES - WEAKNESS - Ankles
- EXTREMITIES - WEAKNESS - Legs - Tendo Achillis

- DREAMS - DIFFICULTIES - journeys, on
- DREAMS - JOURNEYS
- DREAMS - JOURNEYS - China; to
- DREAMS - JOURNEYS - train

- PERSPIRATION - PROFUSE - night
- PERSPIRATION - SUDDEN

- SKIN - DRY
- SKIN - ITCHING
- SKIN - ITCHING - bathing - after
- SKIN - ITCHING - dryness; from
- SKIN - ITCHING - eruptions - without

- SKIN - ITCHING - rubbing - amel.
- SKIN - ITCHING - wool agg.
- GENERALS - AVIATOR'S DISEASE
- GENERALS - INFLAMMATION - Tendons; of
- GENERALS - INJURIES - rupture - Tendons, of
- GENERALS - INJURIES - Tendons, of
- GENERALS - TRAVELLING - ailments from
- GENERALS - WEAKNESS - heat - sun; of the - agg.
- GENERALS - WEAKNESS - vertigo; with

Index

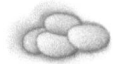

Bibliography

- Dr. John Feltwell: The Story of Silk, Great Britain, 1990, ISBN 0-86299-611-2
- May R. Berenbaum: Blutsauger, Staatsgründer, Seiden-fabrikanten, Germany, 2004, ISBN 3-8274-1519-5
- Margarete Payer: Entwicklungsländerstudie, Teil 1, Kapitel 8: Tierische Produktion, 9. Seidenraupen, 2001, www.payer.de/entwicklung/entw0891.htm
- Silk lexicon of the silk spinnery Plauen, Germany www.spinnhuette.de
- History of Silk, www.silk-road.com
- Chinese Cultural Studies, http://acc6.its.brooklyn.cuny.edu
- Silk, Silk moth, www.wikipedia.org
- Från tekopp till bindtråd, www.rackelhanen.se/swe/1080.htm
- Shenet-Silkeslarv, www.shenet.se/vaxter/silkesmask/html
- Homeopath Renate Siefert: Der Weg der Homöopathie Germany 2016, ISBN 978-3-89060-695-8
- Jeremy Sherr: Dynamics and Methodology of Homeo-pathic Provings, German edition 1998, ISBN 3-933760-00-3

- Patricia Le Roux: Schmetterlinge in der Homöopathie, Germany, 2012, ISBN 978-3-939931-99-7
- Shukla, Herrick, Kohlrausch, Müller: Sieben Schmetterlinge, Deutschland, 2002
- Melissa Assilem: Muttermittel in der Homöopathie, Germany, 2016, ISBN 978-3-941706-92-7
- Dr. Tinus Smits: : Inspiring Homeopathy, Netherlands, German edition, 2015, ISBN 978-90-76189-49-9

Sourcing the homeopathic remedy

Sericum coconum bombyx mori (ser-coc)

Gudjons Apotheke (Augsburg, Germany)
Inh. Dr. (Univ. Urbino) Hannes Proeller e.K.
Phone: +49 821 4441000
www.gudjons-apotheke.de

Remedia (Eisenstadt, Austria)
(probably available at the end of 2024)
Team Santé Salvator Apotheke Mag.pharm. M. Müntz KG
https://remedia.at/shop/

Katrin Rabe - my journey to myself

Born 1966 in Leipzig, Germany
Happy childhood in a loving family

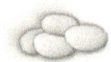

1986-1991	Studying process engineering at Technische Universität Dresden, Germany
1989-2011	Married to Lutz Rabe, two children
1996-2008	Living in Stockholm, Sweden
1999-2006	Project Lead Testlab at Konsumentverket
2001-2004	Studying classical homeopathy under Frans Vermeulen in Stockholm, Sweden
2003-2008	Running own homeopathic practice in Stockholm, Sweden
2005-2007	Basic medical studies at Uppsala University, Sweden
2009	Move back to Germany
2013	Accreditation as Health practitioner (Heilpraktiker), since then running own practice

as homeopath in Leipzig, Germany

Contact the author

Katrin Rabe
KReativ Naturheilpraxis
www.gesund-mit-homöopathie.de
www.kreativ-naturheilpraxis.de
www.katrin-rabe.de

Phone: +49 341 21977535
Mail: katrin@kreativ-naturheilpraxis.de

Advisory/legal disclaimer

The information stated in this book is intended for the study of the homeopathic Materia Medica. The mentioned remedies are not intended for self-medication, but are to be individually adapted to each patient by a qualified healer or therapist.

It is recommended to seek the advice of a homeopathically trained physician or therapist if need be.

All external links were only accessed at time of researching and writing this book. Any later changes by the websites' owners are outside of my control.

Therefore, any liability for external links is excluded.